ALIVE WITH BIPOLAR

By Lorraine Blackburn

'One million people commit suicide every year'
The World Health Organization

Lorraine Blackburn

All rights reserved, no part of this publication may be reproduced by any means, electronic, mechanical photocopying, documentary, film or in any other format without prior written permission of the publisher.

> Published by
> Chipmunkapublishing
> PO Box 6872
> Brentwood
> Essex CM13 1ZT
> United Kingdom

http://www.chipmunkapublishing.com

Copyright © Lorraine Blackburn 2007

Proof-read by Mary Dow

ISBN 978-1-84747-235-9

ALIVE WITH BIPOLAR

BOOK TWO

CHAPTER ONE: THE NORTHERN LIGHTS

It is now two years since I completed my first book, 'There Will Always Be A Sunrise', which, if you have read it, will give you more meaning to this journey. It is mind blowing how much has changed in the past year of my life: it has been a hurricane, pleasant and a calm on the outside, at times, and then at others, I'm stuck in the eye with chaos flying around inside me. My endeavour for this book is to share what has happened in my life because I feel it often helps others to know someone else has been through similar experiences and survived. More then anything I want to pass the fact across that I am still here and surviving and I am even experiencing really happy times and calmness of mind and that my body is resting. It's all new really and I can vividly bring to mind the feelings of anxiety and depression. I really appreciate the days without them, although I still get times when their claws are snagged against my skin and squeezing my mind. I'm not going to enter into great detail here but my life has taken some extreme ups and downs, including another hospital admission in the private hospital, only for ten days this time, and a couple in the NHS hospital. I hope to delve deeper into my feelings this time as people have asked about this from my last book. I think it was harder last time, due to the length of time passed, the fact that my memories were heavily sedated ones and my feeling that I didn't want to bore the reader!!!! So, although I'm a little scared of exposing myself to such an extent, I want this book to be a passage to my thoughts and feelings and that it will have a raw element to it. I've joined an alcoholic support group and I find that when another is sharing their story it can be extremely powerful, bringing goose pimples to my skin, but also tremendously supporting and encouraging;

after all it is very soothing to know you're not alone and others have been there.

So I will tell you where I am now to start your interest into this book. I'm sitting in my rented house where I live with my two children and dog. I have a part time job, am still driving and am excited at the possibility of starting to work for my publishing company. If only the journey to this point had been as simple as that paragraph was to write!!

What is my desire for others to accomplish from this? To see how I've dealt with and learnt from dire situations, to share a common ground and empathy and to grow from how I've learnt to live with my bipolar illness. From my heart I want others to know that we who have mental health illness are living, breathing individuals with thoughts, feelings and we are intelligent and creative. More then anything I want the being that has such issues in life to know they can survive, they can be happy, successful and loved. If I can do it, anyone can, I've pulled myself back up, fought the system and survived. I'm worth it, you're worth it; don't give up, there is light at the end of the tunnel, I know, I've been there, and, although it may not always be constant, it is beautiful and worth the visit like the northern lights. Stay with me.

ALIVE WITH BIPOLAR

CHAPTER TWO: A YEAR ON

It is now nearly a year since my last private hospital admission and guess what? Yet again I'm sitting in the comfy chair in my room over looking the grounds of the hospital. And before you presume that all my words in my previous book were bullshit, they are not. Instead the reader needs to digest this chapter whilst I take them through the passage of the past year of my life since finishing my first book.

My world has changed so drastically it is hard to find a point to start from. Although I must say I am in no surprise to find myself in this room - that is often the usual progression for my condition, i.e. numerous and frequent hospital admissions. I knew a year ago, I'd be spending life under the all encompassing shadow of Bipolar Disorder. I just don't think I realised how hard it is to cohabit with it and to actually accept that my mood can't be stabilized through sheer will power and determination alone (but that definitely helps). Shit it's a steep learning curve!

So I will try to describe the events and experiences, however my mind is currently racing top speed and my concentration is dire so, dare say, this will need editing, although it will give you a greater incite into the magnitude of this illness! I am currently known as having rapid cycling Bipolar Disorder, which basically means I will have at least four or more prominent episodes, a year, of mania or depression. Apparently this is a harder form of manic depression to stabilise. If, as in my current case, you turn the illness up to another level, then you will find an individual in a state of mixed moods. This basically means my mood is alternating at a rapid pace between high and low emotions even within the hour. And believe me it is bloody hard writing in this state whilst simultaneously making any sense.

ALIVE WITH BIPOLAR

I feel as though I've been possessed by demons again, although I am having frequent antipsychotic drugs to help relieve the symptoms. The main cause of this relapse is apparently due to the tremendous amount of stress I've been under for the past six months, which I will discuss. I've been told that a healthy person would also be feeling unwell due to stress, it's just that in my case the Bipolar Disorder has become unstable. I've also had recent bouts of illness where I have been unable to take my medications and/or become dehydrated. These factors have all combined and resulted in me having poor sleep and eating patterns. So, in all, I've lost the plot, and everything I shouldn't have been doing has happened!

Now I'm not sure if I'll include this bit but as I seem to be in quite a prolonged mixed state, i.e. it's been progressively creeping up on me over the past hour, I thought I would try and describe it to you. As I'm writing this the thoughts in my head are racing so fast and way beyond the speed that I'm having trouble keeping up with with my pencil. However I keep finding that I don't know the word I need, and am not aware of the word going down on paper, nor can I read the one I've just written. If I try to reread the paragraphs I've just written the words are purely symbols without meaning, and do not register in my brain. Let us hope that when this episode passes I will be able to find some useful sentences out of the scribbled notes.

As for the rest of my body and mind, they feel like stars spinning out of control from space. I want to stand up and scream and rejoice but also, some how, I want to aggressively cry to the world as well. I can't work out if I'm seeking death or searching for enjoyment and pleasure. I have a really strong desire to strip naked and run, at a hundred miles an hour, around the ward or in the grounds. However I know I'm logical enough to maintain enough control not to. Although that type of release could make me feel a lot calmer!! This might seem full of humour and fun but it's not, in fact I feel exhausted and in desperate painful conflict. As the exhaustion creeps in, my mind releases a tiny gap during which I am able to see how pitiful I've become. As this travels through the cracks and crevasses I am overwhelmed by anger.

I feel desperate to be a character in a horror movie so that I can have the tools and strength to tear out my heart to diminish the pain. I want to grow blades instead of fingers to shred my tormented body to pieces, then to smash my head against the wall until my brain becomes merely pulp. So I guess this can be classified as a wish for self harm, and instead I stay seated trembling all over.

I've been given another dose of an anti-psychotic drug and I can now begin to feel the muscles in my body relaxing, relief yes, in a way, but not from my thoughts yet. As the calm ascends I am becoming painfully aware of what manic and overwhelming levels my thoughts had reached. The sadness snakes its way in, slipping through all the blood vessels of my body and soul. I'm filled with torment and fly questions of why me? And what have I done to deserve this? I just can't see the point of living like this any more, and feel too tired to keep up the fight for survival. Death becomes the ultimate attraction. All my senses are raw and I feel exhausted and utterly spent, apart from a tiny portion, which is now searching for ways and means of killing myself and ending this living nightmare. I know I can't end it all in hospital, I'm being observed too closely for that, but I think of the possibilities for when I get out again. My brain is now becoming calmer and tiny splinters of rest and peace are snaring my body and thoughts. So for now I may be able to relax within my being although I feel highly sensitive to all stimuli.

I have been ill again since then but I will include a previous extract from before that:

Now when I reread this 6 months on it seems a million miles away. I am finally classified as stable, with my emotions centred, void of all extremes. However I remember that time so vividly – the pain, the fear, the helplessness. It is so hard to try to explain to a 'normal' healthy person what these times are like, after all it only seems suited to a horror movie and not reality. I feel a failure and guilty as to why I couldn't control my own emotions without medication, but ultimately I feel fear knowing peace will be short lived in this state.

Being possessed like that made me feel I would never recover or reach the place of one of my favourite sayings- to feel comfortable in my own skin again. This is proof though, because I am again. If you are experiencing this horrendous pain or watching a loved one suffering take comfort from these words. Although we need to take special care of ourselves, as we ARE special individuals, our symptoms can calm down, the pendulum can swing to a lesser degree and we can live satisfying and fulfilling lives. Read on.

ALIVE WITH BIPOLAR

CHAPTER THREE: ANOTHER EPISODE

As I have already mentioned, I have, since my last private hospital admission, had another manic episode. So, before I go into what had been going on in my life, I will discuss what happened. I picked up really quickly after hospital and by the time the summer was round I was really well. I had a boyfriend, was a member of AA's, working extra shifts for my sister and really enjoyed being with the children. We even went on a two-week camping holiday to Dorset and all of us had a fantastic time. So there was nothing wrong with my life, I was not only alive with Bipolar but was actually living a healthy life. So there was no reason for a relapse apart from the Bipolar itself.

It was slow to start off with, the old feelings of racing crept their way in, and I just tried to control them quietly. Then I would become over excited, finding it hard to settle for sleep and wanting to stay up all night. My eating during the day trailed off and then, wham, I started spending big time, always with excuses and in secret. I told my doctor I was going again and he raised my tablets and told me to take a week of bed rest with no stimulus, but this proved impossible with two young children.

By the following Friday I had lost the plot and my Dr wanted to admit me, but I couldn't go to the private hospital as my health insurance no longer covered me. So the only option was St James'. I tried the Navy for funding, but all they did was try to take my children into the care of my then estranged in laws, via social workers and the police. Thankfully I knew none of this, otherwise I would have exploded and I deeply thank my family who all pulled together to stop it. So, after a lot of anguish, I agreed to go into hospital just for a couple of days to have an Eccuvase injection and sleep it off which should have stopped the manic phase.

So I headed off to hospital with my heart in my boots at 8.30pm with my uncle. Just going to the grounds made my stomach sink and entering the building brought back so many awful memories. By this point my body and head were racing but I felt exhausted. I spent most of the time outside, talking with my uncle, while we were waiting for the on call doctor to arrive and there was another patient to be seen before me. Inevitably I reached the stage where I was hallucinating but I didn't let on to the security guards or my uncle. I could see different types of domestic rabbits creeping up the corridor so the others wouldn't see them, but they were all watching me and sending me the message that I was wicked. When I went outside I could see angels sitting in the trees just staring down at me but completely silent.

Lorraine Blackburn

A doctor and a nurse eventually saw me about 12.30 am. I only agreed to stay in if they gave me the injection, which they refused until I was assessed over night. I got very shitty and angry which ended up with me mouthing off to them both. I was promptly told that if I didn't stay that night or the following day I would be sectioned so I had no choice. So I said good-bye to my uncle and headed off to the ward. I guess it had to be that way as I was obsessed with images of slicing my body up and had already sliced my arm.

I was impressed with the ward; it was modern and clean with en-suite shower, single rooms. I was given heavily sedating drugs and, in the end, ordered off to bed as I was too manic. The next day I was given the injection but not in a high enough dose, so I didn't sleep for the three days as planned; instead I was up and about with my mania in the afternoon but was given extra drugs. By Monday I refused to stay any longer and said if they didn't let me go I'd walk. I left with an appointment to see the NHS consultant on the Wednesday, which I did go to and he agreed to discharge me. To be honest, I remember very little of that week as I was so drugged; I was on Lorazepam, Halloperidol, Diazepam, Zimovane and all my normal Bipolar drugs. I lost my boyfriend that week with no explanation other than that he couldn't handle my illness despite all the previous promises.

In all it has taken a long time to get over this episode. I think it was because I wasn't given a strong enough injection. My private doctor said next time he will treat me in the community and I will have to go to Mum's to sleep it off, while she takes care of the children, but he needs a family meeting to discuss what would happen but this hasn't occurred yet. I've got to see the NHS psychiatrist next week and I hope it's not going to be a case of too many chefs spoil Lorraine's broth.

Lorraine Blackburn

I want to high light though that I have got through it. My drugs are being changed and I can hope they will stop the next episode. I still have hope and I can live with this illness, I have to.

ALIVE WITH BIPOLAR

CHAPTER FOUR: LIFE CHANGES

Now I need to journey back to my first book so I can describe the changes. In 'There Will Always Be A Sunrise' I talk of my relationship with Dan, my husband, and how our marriage was set on solid foundations. Well this appears not to have been the situation and in hindsight I believe I wasted too many years trying to convince myself otherwise. If I look back over the previous two years I can see I fought so hard to make our partnership work. I relentlessly tried to re-establish communications between us but Dan would only make a token gesture at trying and then would resort back to his silent self.

I wrote countless letters in an attempt to reach him; I even flew out to Gibraltar alone to see him, which was a major challenge for me. I tried to take an interest in his hobbies, support him in his career and plan time for us to be alone so we could enjoy each other's company. I felt that he was stuck back in the days of St James' Psychiatric Hospital and, although I had made a remarkable recovery and moved on, he had resisted and was stuck fast in those awful memories. Through desperation I suggested marriage guidance and even counselling but he adamantly refused. The only thing we did do together was drink alcohol. My intake was much less then his, but it became a crutch again as I was so unhappy, and this was the only way I could forget. Dan, however, could easily drink three bottles of wine in an evening whilst watching television in silence. Hence we always went to bed at separate times and often awoke to hangovers. As far as I know, his behaviour continues the same.

The lack of communication was the least of my distress though; basically Dan took me through a journey of mental cruelty, bullying me and shredding my self-esteem. He continually told me I was unstable, getting ill and would end up in hospital again. If we had a disagreement those words would be hurled at me, if I was doing something he didn't want me to do those words would be hurled at me, if I was spending, albeit reasonably, those words would be hurled at me, even if I laughed too much those words would be hurled at me!

However, ironically he showed no interest in my condition nor a desire to help me manage it in any way. He would push and push and push until I was teetering on a cliff edge ready to fall into a bottomless pit of insanity. On reflection (as do many others) he was pushing me to the limit in the hope I would crack and become seriously ill again. My only theory for this behaviour is that he would receive more sympathy on leaving me, as he couldn't stay any more, and that way it would be socially understood, in comparison to walking away from a healthy wife that had fought so hard. The only word I can find to describe this is cowardice.

His nature towards me was extremely dominating and he seemed displeased as my independence and strength grew. He bullied me psychologically, criticized me, undermined my confidence and chipped away at my self-esteem. I couldn't possibly explain all the ways here as it would be too extensive and I don't want to waste my words on him. I never received any credit for what I was achieving in life and the hardest attitude of all is that he had zero respect for me, which can be seen in our last night together.

He had spent the day being very cagey about his up and coming travels, and he deflected any attempt that I made to suggest I meet him in Turkey. The plan was to have an early night and spend some quality time together; however all he did was sit and get pissed despite my best efforts to encourage him not to. When we eventually got to bed a row evolved through which I was able to discover the truth of the perceptions he had of me. He told me I wasn't worth anything, I would always be ill, I owed everything to him and because of this he could treat me however he wanted to. I felt disgusted, hurt, cheated, small, pathetic and sickened. How could I ever forget or forgive those words? How could I ever continue in my marriage knowing that was how he truly felt about me?

He went and slept in our son's room on my request whilst I cuddled up with my son in our bed. The next morning he came in, lifted my son back to his bed, then got into ours, laid on top of me and performed sexual intercourse on me. I laid still, desperately wanting him to leave me alone whilst silent tears cascaded down my face. He knew I was crying. He knew I was as rigid as a board and he must of known I was not being a consenting adult, but he continued until he was satisfied, got off me and went and got ready for work.

I don't know how I got through the next hour and a half, trying to keep a clear mind and get the children ready for school, wishing the minutes would pass until he left for Plymouth. He kissed the children goodbye, kissed me on the cheek, went out of the door and, although he didn't realise it then, out of our marriage forever.

I went to my parents that morning and poured out the reality of the situation. They were both very supportive although saddened. The next few months saw drastic changes, which developed steadily. I removed my wedding ring a few weeks later when I discovered he'd been in Scotland but not phoned the children. I wrote to him and told him the marriage was over and I felt he needed psychological help. From that point I went to my solicitors and had to be up front about everything including my illness and this was very hard.

One of the hardest days of my life was telling the children that Mummy and Daddy would no longer be living together. As I sat them down I thought shit, what I'm about to tell them is going to change their precious, safe lives forever. Having that power was extremely frightening, knowing that if I said the wrong thing that could affect their futures, but then whatever I said would be the wrong thing surely?

I can't remember the words I used, but they went running off up the stairs to their rooms shouting and screaming. I tried to follow them but as soon as I was close enough to touch them they would run their separate ways and hide. I left then, for five minutes, to give them some space and then, one at a time, took them in my arms and held them tight whilst they sobbed their broken hearts up to me, their whole bodies shaking. I cried with them and in the end we were all sat on the floor of the lounge crying and sobbing. I think this really helped as, though I was the 'strong' one telling them the news, I could also be the 'strong' one crying with them, holding and being held. I continually said it was okay to cry and I would answer any questions they wanted to ask, and that it wasn't their fault at all.

When the tears eventually stopped we jumped in the car with the dog for a two hour ramble in a secluded wood. I think their emotional energy ricocheted off the tall pine trees whilst they covered themselves in mud pretending to be red Indians. This slice of normality and exercise let them release pent up steam and they bombarded me with questions about Mummy and Daddy. A lot of their queries were very grown up and practical and I was not only amazed at their understanding but also comforted that my honest approach had been the best one.

After warm baths and clean clothes we sat again on the lounge floor tucking into a take away Chinese meal. It was my way of giving them a shared treat without resulting to bribed gifts, and it worked. Later in the week I bought them a soft toy dog each. I told them they were special dogs because if they were feeling sad about Mummy and Daddy and they didn't want to give me a cuddle, they could cuddle their dogs. This has also been very effective as they are a neutral source of comfort and has helped especially if they are confused or want to be on their own. Needless to say they are now firm night time buddies.

So this has been a huge change in my life since my last book. I never imagined it would happen to me as I thought we had been through the worst and everything would have improved. I still think the experience of St James is what damaged our marriage beyond saving, so yet again my illness has caused mayhem in my life. However I am much happier now and this independent life is good; I wouldn't change it now, although I do need to get through the divorce and financial quarrels without sinking- maybe a book three is to come!

When he sees the children Dan seems to have less time for my daughter and this is also reflected in telephone calls. However, on returning home, my son has sobbed in my arms and collapsed on the floor; I've lost count of the numbers of cuddles we've had on the porch floor as Daddy has driven away. So, currently two and a half years on, the picture is one of legalities whilst both sides battle for a satisfactory financial outcome. I still get strong flashbacks and my heart breaks that it has finally come to an end. My emotions are such extremes for Dan, sometimes it's happiness for shared good times, otherwise it's a mixture of sadness and anger but always is the underlying relief of freedom – as that of an albatross flying the crest of the waves and knowing I am now at a peaceful distance.

CHAPTER 5: MOVING ON

If I now retrace my steps back towards the end of the summer three major events occurred which I think were instigators for me in finding a new life for the three of us. First, after I painstakingly mastered the elements of my computer, I printed up and circulated a dozen copies of my finished book. I received many positive and interesting responses but unfortunately the issue of mental health and its survival were not covered by the majority of publishers.

However during a very hectic morning of the school summer holidays, I received a call from Jason Pegler of Chipmunkapublishing. I was unprepared for the call and taken by surprise- whilst my 2 children and dog were having a competition as to who could make the loudest noises whilst simultaneously running around the house!!!! I remember only a few of his questions and, taking into consideration that my daughter disconnected us mid-flow, my answers definitely fell short of my feelings! I do remember one though and my clear answer now would be yes it has been painful to write, I have tortured myself reliving memories, astonished myself by discovering new facts and events in my life, and have cried at times as though my tears would be endless and continue for all eternity. I have found, though, that through writing 'There Will Always Be A Sunrise', I have surprised myself by the vast diversity of strength and coping skills I have displayed. It has also been hugely therapeutic: working through my life by word, by sentence, by chapter and by book. Jason made no promises to me but said it would be reviewed in January for a publication decision to be made.

For me this was like taking a bright yellow highlighter pen and illuminating the word hope every time it was typed in my manuscript! It was as if the word hope had become a pebble tossed into a flat calm sea, making the surrounding circular effect of the water grow outwards and onwards. This gave me the hope that, if my book was to be published, it could help another to survive the torment or could assist an individual in learning about such a socially taboo subject. I played with many thoughts but mainly those of: that maybe I could make a difference and that in some way, no matter how diverse, there would be some meaning to the pain I had gone through in my life. It gave me hope. On a more quirky note, about a month later and some what impulsively, I had a tattoo done on my lower back. It is of a humpback whale, which to me signifies the vastness of the ocean and the freedom this represents, and underneath I had hope written in Celtic letters resembling waves and there is no need for me to explain that one!

ALIVE WITH BIPOLAR

It was also about this time that I started to help Sue out at her new catering business. She was getting it up and running with a business partner and was then leaving in October to travel the world for six months with her husband. I found it really hard when I first started; I was always forgetting things and having to have instructions repeatedly explained. I also had very little confidence and no self esteem, and felt very anxious as I had not worked for nine years. However, with time I found that my memory improved along with my dexterity and initiative. I just needed to be in a safe, supportive environment, amongst people that understood my illness, and the limitations it imposed on me. I guess I've been one of the lucky ones to have experienced it. Once I started to get paid I felt responsibility and the experience that others depended on me. It also gave invaluable structure to my week and regular social exposure, both of which help in mental health. It was great and I was succeeding – something that was never expected of me - after all I was meant to have been institutionalised for the remainder of my life. Dan, needless to say, was not happy with me holding down a job, and continually criticized the so called inadequacies of the other components of my life. He was also very unimpressed by my call from Jason and opposed the possibility of it being published; in fact he has never read it.

I do enjoy my work, but I also know I'm lacking in mental stimulation as it's mainly manual. Don't get me wrong, it can be very satisfying to create a gourmet platter from scratch, but my mind craves rousing and inspiring nourishment. Some days are a real struggle and I can't focus or concentrate, or my anxiety is extreme and I hardly respond to anyone. However I get by, no, those are the wrong words, I do a bloody good job, and can be extremely fast when my mind's racing towards its mania origins!!!!! All it has taken is being given a chance in a supporting and understanding environment- after all creativity is meant to be a bonus of bipolar disorder!!!

Finally I had become close with a male friend. I know our friendship would never have happened if I had been loved and contented within my relationship with Dan. It reached the heady pinnacle of love but to have gone with it and made a new beginning would have caused too much hurt and pain all round. So the sensible and most selfless action that could have been taken was instigated – we parted on our separate ways and left our memories and emotions behind, all be they precious, but never to be revealed again. I do believe, ironically, that I stayed with Dan longer because of this friendship as it was a source of love, companionship and a touching of souls. Without that I could never have suffered and continued with the pain Dan inflicted on me. The memories are treasured and the 'what ifs' are never delved in to; it has now been laid to rest with the few other golden times I have of my life. So it was time to take a more positive action for my new beginning and new life.

ALIVE WITH BIPOLAR

CHAPTER SIX: A DESTRUCTIVE RELATIONSHIP

So I'm back nearly full circle- but I need to discuss another destructive relationship I found myself in. It will help now if you cast your mind back to when I highlighted what one of my professionals said: that is people with bipolar disorder usually attract and become lost in abusive relationships.

After having so much experience of this I can hardly believe I allowed myself to become engulfed in the situation, and I'm only now coming up gasping for air at the end of it. First, Ben was a friend of the family and was described as being caring, trusting, loving, funny, sensitive etc. Mentally I had already left Dan, removing my wedding ring, making my solicitor's appointment etc. So, after swapping texts, I thought ok, let's go out for a friendly drink. So that's how it started and Ben seemed perfect in every way. However as time progressed it was apparent that he had problems, especially relationship issues with having been hurt in the past.

I wasn't concerned, I just thought, well I'm a can of worms with my bipolar disorder, and, full of self importance, I thought I could help him in some way. I'm not going to enter into great details of this friendship as I'm not prepared to allow myself to expend my energy on it. Basically over four months he very gradually turned into a bully, becoming very controlling and domineering whilst continually putting me down. We parted company quite a few times but he some how made me feel guilty and request his forgiveness. This was a complete repeat of Ernie without the physical or sexual abuse.

When we fell out I would be a victim to his continuous phone calls until late at night, and he had even appeared at my house past 11pm one night to shout at me. The calls were always full of threats and of how awful I was and all the problems I had, and they were always full of hate and venom, shouting at me continually. I often found myself trying to say anything to calm him down and dissolve the anger. Every time it happened, the following day he would be oblivious to the hurt and abuse he'd inflicted on me, just carrying on as normal, all kindness and light, without forgetting that it had, after all, been all my fault!!

I think one of the last straws was when I discovered he'd been sitting outside my house at 10pm in his car just watching. I presume he was waiting for a man to emerge or just checking up on me whilst all the time I was in bed. The next day I sent him a nice text explaining I couldn't see him any more as it wasn't helping me or my illness. Almost immediately he was on my doorstep, luckily the children were out and I didn't let him in. Then for about an hour and a half I was subjected to all numerable amounts of abuse through the closed door. Then the phones started ringing and each time I cut him off the other phone rang and so on. I called my close friend and via her advice told him I was going to call the police, but it made no difference to him. I was alone, in the dark, cowering in the corner of the kitchen on the floor, with threatening abuse bombarding me from all directions. He informed me that if he didn't get me that night he would continue to follow me until he did. Eventually, after calling two of my family members, he was convinced to leave, but it was all a nightmare with a lot of astonishment and confusion on all our behalves. As soon as we were on our own again though, the calls and text messages began. The two children, the dog and I all slept in the same room.

ALIVE WITH BIPOLAR

The next few days were awful. I lived off of my nerves, constantly checking over my shoulder, looking out for his car and checking the locks. The children were terrified and became very clingy and emotional. After a few days we exchanged texts but I always refused when he wanted to come round and talk. Then he started calling: it was apologies at first but then anger and blame directed at me. So I think that the amount of anxiety he put me through and, consequently, the severe lack of sleep was enough to tip me over a somewhat already teetering edge into my bipolar, becoming completely unstable, and me being admitted to hospital. Again he was full of apologies and support and kindness, again I forgave him and in a contorted way blamed myself. That is until this week: there has been another episode because I wasn't doing what he expected or things how he wanted them done. I think on the surface his rage was more contained but the words of hate and loathing still illuminated his communications, blaming me for all sorts of nasty thoughts and actions. So this time I have clearly stated I want nothing to do with him whatsoever. If needs be, I will call the Police as he left me with a huge sense of fear. When I look back I can clearly see how he undermined me, chipped away at my confidence, criticized me and controlled my life. So how did I let such a destructive relationship into my life again? I don't have the answer to that. A year on from writing this I have seen him a couple of times and exchanged a few texts but that is all.

ALIVE WITH BIPOLAR

CHAPTER SEVEN: THE NOT SO LONE YACHTSWOMEN

After exchanging information with my consultant and psychologist it was decided that I did need another hospital admission for medication change, re-establishing a routine and a much needed rest. Again various people around me questioned this decision and denied I required admission and said that I would end up in there for weeks. It's very hard, when you're in so much psychological turmoil, to deal with these over sensitive opinions and it requires far too much mental energy to alleviate everyone's fears. I even had a huge row with my dad when he informed me that there was no such thing as bipolar disorder, it was all in my head and I just used it to run away from life and never face up to things. According to him all I did was cause trouble to the family and leave my children. As you can imagine, my anger had no holds and I fought back just as hard, pointing out that it was likely that someone in his family had passed it down to me. Afterwards I realised I should have just quietly asked him why he was on antidepressants, was it 'all in his head' and what was he hiding from?

At this point I need to give some extra information at the request of some of the members of the family, both those that have and have not read my last book. I think that as the likelihood of my book being published drew closer, individuals began to have concerns as to the contents. I will reiterate that I have written this from the heart and as the truth on how I viewed and experienced events. So basically I need to make the other side of my relationship with my dad clearer and that the agro was not all from his location but mine as well. Apparently I was a difficult child but even more so as a teenager – continually having tempers, sulks and exploding at the smallest of things. Having spoken to my family recently they believed it was premenstrual tension alone; until now that is, when everyone can see how this could have been my illness manifesting in its early stages.

So I was a highly strung teenager, learning to escape using alcohol whilst coming to loggerheads with a dominant and strict father who was a self medicating alcoholic. Basically the outcome of this was a frequent clashing of minds. So it wasn't all his fault; we were both very strong characters and both spoke our minds, so by my standing up to him we had numerous arguments, meeting head long in the middle, with neither of us backing down. I also believe that our personalities were of such extremes that we constantly collided. I still find it hard to forgive and forget. A classic example is this debate that bipolar disorder doesn't exist. When I tried to be understanding and to help him grasp my illness I suggested that he read some of the literature my mum had been given; his response to me was that it was all a load of rubbish and he would not read it!

However this is where it gets very confusing for me because my emotions are at the two extremes of love and dislike. Whilst I've been in hospital for this stay he has bent over backwards, helping in any which way possible. He's taken and collected my children from their school, he's entertained them, loved them and supported them. This has mainly been done alone as my mum has been working extra shifts at work to cover my absence and my dad has been doing the long round work trip twice a day without a whisper of complaint. In response to this it is obvious and clear to see that my children adore him and vice versa. My mum has also been super-woman, keeping everything working whilst balancing the tricky schedule she is under. I cannot begin to describe the love, affection and support my parents have shown me, especially in the past few months. This has been unconditional. So I can honestly say my heart is full of love and thanks to them both. A year down the line since writing this I can say there is a definite calm between my dad and I, we have common ground at last and we've stopped arguing, he is always helping me out in all sorts of ways and we share a lot of laughter. Does he understand my illness more? I think so as he's had to get use to it but he is especially proud now I'm coming off a lot of my medication, but that's another tale for another book!

I explained to the children in our normal way why I had to go into hospital for a while. Again we had an in depth discussion into my chemicals! This time I had to explain they were moving between happy and sad and that the changes were occurring up to six times an hour. My daughter without clarity of reason could already see this was happening and they both understood it had to become level again. They also grasped that because they were changing so quickly I was very tired. So in their simple logic they realised that I needed my tablets changing so my chemicals and therefore moods could 'sit' in the middle and that I needed a good rest. I hated leaving them but it makes it less painful knowing they understand.

ALIVE WITH BIPOLAR

CHAPTER EIGHT: RETURN TO THE PRIVATE HOSPITAL

I found my hospital stay more frustrating this time, and I was also extremely frightened. My consultant was fantastic, promising to be with me every step of the way and not leaving me. The episode I've described at the beginning of this book is pretty much how I felt the majority of the time. I did manage to get to two therapy groups but I found both upsetting as my thoughts were pretty selfish. I kept thinking everyone else had a more than decent chance of recovery whereas my illness was for life and it depressed me. All I kept thinking was 'yeah great, I'll be patched up and discharged until the next episode and so on'.

I don't think I was exactly depressed in my first week at the hospital, it was more of a case that my thoughts were racing top speed and were becoming quite bizarre. I also had a reaction to an antipsychotic drug I'd been given and my whole body shook violently. The nurses even had to place my tablets in my mouth and hold the cup to my lips so I could swallow them down with water. If I tried to take a drink myself I would miss my face and it would take both my hands to place the cup down on the table against an unseen force.

There were also quite a few screw ups on my medication, and, since my St James' experience, I insist I know what I'm taking and when and what the side effects are. I think this was the door that was left ajar for the paranoia and suspicion to slip in. Due to the shaking I didn't want to leave the room, and it was impossible trying to eat. I also had a second experience of hallucinations at this point. I was sitting on my bed and saw three cats walk quite calmly and in no obvious hurry across the floor of my room. They were crystal clear to me, all were on the heavier side and one was white and ginger,

ALIVE WITH BIPOLAR

one was black, and one was a mixture. I knew logically they couldn't have been there but they were so real I believed I could reach out and touch them. They left through the closed window not jumping and smashing it to splinters but instead just flowing through the glass.

This was obviously distressing and for once I pressed the nurse call bell. She was lovely and went to great efforts to explain how there was no way any cats could be in my room or the hospital and that I was safe. What I was more frightened about was not the reality of the cats or that they could hurt me, but the actuality that I knew I was hallucinating and what the fuck was happening to my mind. I didn't get any answers so I tried to settle down again. Then out of the corner of my eye I thought I saw some 'things' moving; when I looked over at my comfy armchair I could see that it was swarming in black ants – thousands of them. It was as though the chair was no longer an inanimate object, but instead wriggling and moving of its own accord. So yet again I was comforted and reassured but my fear didn't lie with the cats or the ants but with my mind and how obviously sick it was, and out of my control. The next day my room was moved nearer to the nurses' station as the 'really sick' patients weren't allowed to be that far up the corridor.

The final situation, which led to my leaving hospital earlier than the advice I was given, began on a Sunday. I actually woke up feeling depressed and suicidal and I couldn't shake it off. One of the nurses had been especially supportive throughout the day to me. I went for a half hour walk to try and shake off the feelings, but all I could think about was killing myself and I walked round and round the hospital to see if I could jump off the roof. Apparently, on my return, I discovered I was just about to have someone go out and look for me. As the afternoon progressed

ALIVE WITH BIPOLAR

I became increasingly suspicious, paranoid and suicidal. I reached the stage where my body language was withdrawn and I was almost mute. I wanted to put my wardrobe in front of the door to stop 'them' from coming in but it was too heavy. I had been given Librium throughout the day but it hadn't helped. I kept stating that each time I was given more.

Eventually I sat on a pillow, on the floor, arms around my knees and rocking rhythmically. I had made a barrier around me of chairs, the bed and the table; and put jugs etc on the table so I couldn't be seen over from the door. Each time they left the door open I closed it. I was frightened and believed they were out to get me. I wasn't scared they would hurt me but I just knew I must not communicate with or let them come near me. I didn't want to trick them into keeping me alive. When the nurse I was friendly with asked me what I was doing on the floor I barely whispered that I was safer there as I couldn't fall off. The on call GP was contacted and I was given more Librium and a different prn that my consultant knew wasn't working for me. I eventually begged for help as the drugs weren't touching me and I stated it was unethical to leave me in this state, I was terrified and paranoid.

When he eventually turned up he stood on the other side of the room, which in itself was intimidating as I was curled up on the floor. I couldn't understand his accent or hear what he was saying clearly. Again I pointed out how unethical it was to leave me in such anguish to which he promised to write me up and give me something to help alleviate the feelings. I waited and waited until eventually the night medications came around, only for me to discover he hadn't written me up for anything then or throughout the night. Did anyone care? I'd been up front with them; why weren't they honest and no bullshit with me? If I could have willed myself to death then I would have done. Consequently I was up frequently throughout the night. When I did eventually get washed and dressed I thought fuck it, if they're not going to help me I'll do it myself, and headed off for a walk in the grounds with the Darkness blasting in my ears. After about five minutes I felt a hand on my shoulder and was informed I had to return to the ward immediately, as I was on ten minute observations and wasn't allowed in the grounds alone. I put up a verbal fight with lots of fucks and how come I was yesterday and how was I meant to get better on my own.

I was marched back to the ward and I slammed my door so hard I am still surprised it didn't fall off the hinges. I had a smoke and calmed down a little before I got in touch with my outpatient psychologist. He came straight over and listened to my some what bemused account of events and said he'd get the consultant to see me, but also gave me reassurance that he was at the end of the phone if I needed him. When I first returned from my walk the staff brought in some drugs for me to take. I was distressed but still asked what they were and almost felt forced into taking them. Once they'd gone I realised it had only been more Librium and an extra dose of my antipsychotic drug which had no effect as a prn drug. My thoughts were clear: if it wasn't helping me then I would not take it pointlessly or to satisfy a belief that the 'appropriate' action had been taken by the staff! So I went to the toilet and forced my fingers down my throat and vomited it all up. I did admit this to both my psychologist and consultant when I saw them. I wanted the message to be put across that I was still in charge of myself and would be active within my nursing and medical care. In all honesty I must admit now that paranoia came in to play a great part as I was convinced that the staff were out to get me and sedate me despite their reassurances!

So by 2pm I had packed my bags, successfully achieved my goals and had nagged the staff to ring him at 3.15 pm. The reply was I would still have to wait until 4pm for the decision!! I was eventually released on time with medications and out patient appointments but sadly and truthfully I didn't leave with a definite farewell, just that I hoped it would be longer before I saw them all again.

So here I am, now back home with my children and dog, but not at work yet, I'm still leaving it another week. I think I feel confused really, strong that I have got through another episode, especially that I was aware enough to know that I had become psychotic. It was always the voice in my head poisoning me but some how I was detached from it. I recognised the sound, however the words were illogical but equally compelling. When I was alone with my racing thoughts I was convinced I was being attacked from all sides by all the nursing staff. As far as I believed their aim was to transform me into a zombie so I could be locked away forever.

I also felt I wanted to tear myself apart limb by limb, to destroy all the torturing sensations and tormenting emotions. So again my ultimate goal was death, because with death I believed I would have peace. My state of exhaustion was also a formidable force against me. It was all encompassing both physically and mentally. I didn't even find relief at night as my dreams were horrifying or I was a million miles from attaining sleep. Again my GP, psychologist and consultant have been outstanding as have the majority of the nursing staff.

ALIVE WITH BIPOLAR

I can't really say where I am at this point in my life. I know ahead of me there is more stress due to my divorce. I am also only too clearly aware that this illness is not stable and straight forward for me. Also, at the moment I will admit it's bloody hard and in hindsight I agree with the medical staff that I left hospital too early. I have learnt a lot about my own strengths again and also how painfully open my weaknesses are. I think one of the most frightening facts I have ever learnt about this illness is that beyond a certain point I have no logical control despite all my desperate and searching intellectual efforts. At some point I now know I will have to realise the truth, place my trust in my carers and allow them to treat me with their medications no matter what the strength. This terrifies me but I will have to deal with it over and over again, and at times will have to compromise my independence to them.

However, on a positive note, there is a lot to look forward to. Relationship-wise I have the freedom to meet and spend time with a person that can understand my illness, to have an equal friendship and most importantly to share a lot of laughter. I no longer have to settle for abuse and second best because I have an illness; instead I have the equal opportunity for happiness. I'm also leading an independent life, am holding down a job, being the major carer for my children and maintaining a safe and happy home for them. Finally, the crest of the wave for me is that my book is to be published by chipmunkapublishing. I have signed the contract and although we're a while away from finalities, I feel as though I have achieved something strong, invaluable and even guiding. Just by writing it I have given myself hope alongside understanding and I believe I will be able to pass on these feelings to others. I am unsure of my future but no doubt it could always

ALIVE WITH BIPOLAR

lead to a further sequel of 'There Will Always Be A Sunrise'!!

CHAPTER NINE: RELATIONS

Well I seem to have managed to squeeze in another chapter all down to the fact of my failed relationships. After the traumatic previous one, and all the stuff with Dan I decided not to get involved for a while and this was also around the same time I started Alcoholics Anonymous.

I went through a tearful meeting one night and one of my fellow recoverers called me outside and gave me a big hug. It just went from there really, started with texts, then the phone calls until we eventually met up in secret. We kept the relationship very much on the quiet as it is frowned upon in early recovery. However, as our feelings grew so did our confidence and we laid it open that we were a couple.

We got on very well as best friends do, and he became extremely close to my children; it was as if we were a family unit again. We even had a fantastic camping holiday in Dorset doing loads of things such as star gazing, fair ground rides, rock pooling to river boating. It was great and we were all happy and contented.

Once we got back he was tied up with family affairs and I got back into the flow of work and the children; the only problem was the swing bit- it was creeping off course again. I let it go free for one week end just to make sure and then phoned my consultant. I was prescribed a week in a darkened room with no stimuli and a drug increase. However I think it was too late as I became over happy, racing in my conversation, going on spending sprees and was up throughout the night building stools and attempting to cook dinner. By the end of the week I was into it fully. My doctor said I had to be admitted and have an Accuvase injection to knock me out for three days and get my natural clock back. The main problem was I had no private health care left – I tried every which way to raise the money, even the Navy, but that didn't work. I was to find later that this was a mistake as they involved social workers and the next morning my family, including my boyfriend, had to go through all sorts of dilemmas to stop the children being taken by my in laws. So at 8.30pm I kissed my kids goodbye and headed off to the NHS hospital after many calls organising it.

I never thought I would be a patient there again and with the emotional support of my uncle we climbed the large steps to the hospital. It took three hours to be seen; the majority of the time I was chain smoking or I was cutting my already split arm with an earring as I just wanted to release the misery inside me. I also thought I could see angels in the trees and rabbits in the corridors. I told the doctor I would not be admitted unless I had the injection straight away which wasn't possible so we compromised on

ALIVE WITH BIPOLAR

Halloparadol and Lorazepam until the following day. She also told me that although I was an informal patient at the moment she could and would section me at any time. My uncle saw me off and I was shown to my bedroom, at least it was a single room with a shower and no dormitories as before. I was given my medication and was still flying around until I got sternly told to go to bed by one of the nurses.

I actually managed to sleep all night, and then took the courage to face the rest of the ward. It was modern and new but the characters were duplicates; I even saw an old face from before. I just kept on until they gave me my injection; I wasn't wiped out as I had hoped or as they had envisaged but just kept on having naps and getting up for a fag. It was so boring in there and although the staff were friendly, I didn't experience any one to one time with them. By Monday morning I'd had enough and I told them if I didn't get discharged I'd do it myself. In the end I settled for home leave and back to see the consultant on Wednesday. When I saw him he wanted me to stay on the Lorazepam and the Halloparadol and consider staying NHS.

So back to the relationship side; what my boyfriend was left with by Thursday night was a doped up vegetable. I didn't realise this as I was just doing what the doctor told me, but saying that I did decide to stop my tablets myself on the Friday as I didn't feel right. So my boyfriend avoided me Friday and cancelled our arrangements, he then told me Saturday he needed space from us, and by Monday had put the keys through the door and had taken his belongings. He's here now whilst I'm writing in the garden; he's in the new house painting and avoiding me like the plague. The only explanation that he has is that he can't handle my illness, he just can't do it. This amazes me as I was only really bad for about seven to ten days, and we had discussed it before and he'd learnt a lot about it. Shit, what if he'd experienced one of my depressions??! I am sad we are apart and I will miss him and it will be very hard on the children, but this goes deeper for me. How will I ever find a man that will love me enough to cope with my disorder? I don't think I will and this leaves me so sad I could split in two. It's not just about him but the whole picture too. It's courageous to say you will stand by someone when life is easy, but to run away when it's tough is weak and cruel. Ok he said he could not cope but he should not have made those un-kept promises and given me false hope. But it is ok because I am coping, I've got my children and a future, albeit uncertain, so I will continue to hope for serenity and peace in body and soul whether I stay on my own or not.

Now for my relationship with my dad, this is an update really. It's changed!! He has been very loving, caring and supportive. He helps with the children from doing home work to helping disciplining to just giving me time out. We can now talk about issues without wages and I can really get good advice off of him and he's always doing things to help me. We hardly ever have any arguments and if we do they are short lived and more like bantering. My dad also helps me out financially at family functions, where if he didn't we wouldn't be able to take part, so I'm eternally grateful. The way I see things now is I've laid the past to rest. I love my dad and admire him most of the time!

CHAPTER TEN: A PARTNER OF A LIFE TIME – ALCOHOL

Well I've finally decided to be honest enough and admit the full relationship I've had with alcohol. Basically I'm a recovering alcoholic and have known since I was fourteen that I had a problem with the demon drink. However it is not until now that I'm thirty-six, I can admit it freely.

As you already know my dad use to drink and alcohol was a strong component in that side of the family. I can remember getting drunk at New Year parties in my early teens, and around fourteen years old I went to a friend's instead of guides and got plastered, only to be delivered unconscious to my sisters; luckily my mum and dad were out.

Then as my mood swings crept in, mainly depression, and after watching my dad nightly, I decided that maybe alcohol could be my solution. When everyone was in bed I would creep downstairs and take numerous swigs from each bottle – it didn't matter which as long as I got the sting factor and, after, numbness, so on occasions I would be at school drunk. As I progressed onto college these sessions became more frequent.

So I would be without sleep and pissed and that is how I sat my A-level finals. Alcohol had already become my main coping mechanism and the behaviour of secret drinking was established. When I started my nurse training in Bath and started socialising and going to pubs and clubs, I found my new tipple was cider, normally seven pints a throw, and it beat the taste of the mixed drinks cabinet. Although the other girls would go out, I soon realised that they didn't drink as much as me or pile up drinks at closing time, desperate to get as much in as possible. I also started to have cans and bottles of cider alone in my room, hidden away in case anyone knocked on my door, and I know no one else was doing this secret solo drinking.

I quite often had black outs and didn't remember coming home or who had come home with me; I think I felt so wretched I just didn't care. I know I was on occasions still drunk when at work in the mornings; I got away with it by saying I had a hangover rather than that I was drunk. When I was high I would go out every night and get into these states as there was always some acquaintance I could go out with.

I shudder at the danger of it now, as, when like that, I had no sense of safety nor of whom I was with, and may have ended up in the wrong hands or with the police. One night I had a psychotic phase mixed with alcohol and walked bare foot in my pyjamas to town and then all through the streets. How did I get away with it?

Lorraine Blackburn

When I left Bath my drinking slowed for a bit in the amounts but I would still have to drink every night. Once I started at university it was basically a free for all as if I had a valid passport to drink as much as I wanted, whenever I wanted, in pubs, clubs, the student union and of course at home alone; after all I was a mature student. Yet again I put myself in danger, wandering home, completely pissed, on my own. I always seemed to be drinking the most, taking it on beyond reasonable limits. I knew I had a problem but I decided I was too young to have to worry about it and made goals for when I would stop but I never did. I would also go without food so I could afford my alcohol.

Around this time I got heavily into the yachting scene and was introduced to the nectars of wine, champagne and wild parties – I was having a ball. I could say I was well re my bipolar but I don't think that's true, more of a case of a manic episode- but I loved it. I also met my husband, a naval officer and a heavy drinker himself. Our social life was the pub, drunken dinner parties and getting pissed at home on wine and cider. After he went to sea, my home solo drinking shot up and I would be a regular at my corner shop for booze.

Throughout my life with Dan we spent most nights drunk, only missing alcohol if our hangovers were too severe. The only period I had in my life when my alcohol intake was low was when I sailed across the Pacific ocean, but when we got to shore I made up for it ten times over. I was reasonably controlled during my pregnancies but as soon as I got home from hospital I wanted alcohol. I drank through my two episodes of post natal depression to try and take the pain and confusion I was feeling away. When we moved to Plymouth I hit a manic phase and drank like a fish, partying every night and getting tangled up in an affair.

At this stage in my life I entered a phase of spending most of it in hospital. I was in and out of it in Plymouth and spent over a year in Portsmouth. Despite going through detox every time I was discharged or on leave, I went straight back to drinking. I know it sounds crazy but I'm an alcoholic and when we're addicted that's what we do.

It wasn't until I was newly diagnosed at thirty-four as having bipolar disorder, and in the private hospital for the first time, that I came across Alcoholics Anonymous face to face. I had gone through a detox in hospital and this absolutely stunning woman came to speak to me; I couldn't believe she was an alcoholic and was shocked when she said so!! So I was discharged sober, made all the right phone calls to AA and made all the right noises but didn't actually go. I don't know why exactly, I think I was worried it would be "gody" and I felt I could do it all on my own. How wrong I was; I lasted just three months.

    I spent the next year drinking, feeling guilty and nodding but not hearing when my consultant told me I must not drink. In retrospect I think I was in self-destruct mode and it must have been horrible for my children to watch. I drank every night, alone, normally wine; once I had rushed the kids off to bed so I could open my bottle. I know my daughter has seen me in numerous stages of inebriation, sometimes putting me to bed, and I would have the all too familiar blackouts. I was trapped by day, agitated and wracked with guilt, by night desperate for a drink to take my feelings away – it was just a continual cycle. I would have hangovers and sleep a lot of the day so I was never organised or in control of my life. What a way to lead a life and goodness knows what effect it was having on my bipolar illness and my family.

Then one day was different, although it started out the same. In the early evening I finished off my first bottle of wine and then walked the children down to the corner shop to buy a second. When we got back, the children were playing out the front whilst I was gulping my wine, when I realised I didn't want to do it anymore. I had a strong compulsion to phone AA which I did, and they were brilliant being very supportive and encouraging. They arranged for a lady to take me to a meeting on the Monday and asked me not to drink the following day. When I woke up Sunday I had this sensation of freedom which was fantastic after all these years.

So here I am, six months into the fellowship and my life has changed beyond recognition. For me the main benefit I feel is the love and

ALIVE WITH BIPOLAR

friendship I am welcomed by as I enter the rooms. There is so much sobriety and wisdom I always leave full of new advice and help. Even the new comer is able to contribute. I had a slip up last week and took a sip of wine, but once I shared it at the meeting, amongst my friends and with their support, I left with even more strength and resolve and without criticism. I now have a higher power, not god, but a guidance I trust in and hand my life over to. It's amazing at times how my higher power comes through for me. I also have numerous numbers I can call, any time of the day or night, and, if they can, they will be there for me. The back-bone of the fellowship is the twelve steps that you work at and travel through. I'm still on the beginning ones but working them each day helps to give me peace and serenity. My sponsor is fantastic, she listens to me and very subtly helps to guide me in the right direction; I would be lost without her.

Lorraine Blackburn

The only thing I will quote out of AA is The Serenity Prayer as it means so much to me and I try to follow it everyday:

> God grant me the serenity to accept
> The things I cannot change
> Courage to change the things I can
> And the wisdom to know the difference.

So here I am now, doing step one again but feeling positive as I have so many people behind me. So all I can say is if you think you have an alcohol problem then phone AA as you will find the help and it works!!

Since first writing this chapter time has moved on and I am now twenty months sober and I do it by not taking that first drink and staying sober one day at a time.

ALIVE WITH BIPOLAR

CHAPTER ELEVEN: A SHORT ONE

Well I seem to have had a couple of weeks' grace, where I felt pretty good after my manic episode, thinking that the worst was over and great, no problems. However last Sunday I woke in the depths of depression, I had phoned my doctor on the Friday knowing it was coming on but I couldn't locate him.

So how have I felt? As though I have wanted the world to swallow me up and take me away from my misery. I've had no energy to do anything and all I have done is sleep all day. One thing that has helped is going to AA's; otherwise I know I would have drank. Another practise that has eased the pain is talking to my higher power, I don't mean god, I mean the higher power I have handed my alcohol over to and this time my depression. I have been more honest with others about the turmoil I've been going through but it's been hard as my dad is in hospital.

The most shocking thing is that at times I've wished for my children to just not be, so I can go ahead and kill myself; so again you can see how my children literally keep me alive at times like this. I don't want this to be a long chapter or to dwell on it as it has been less then a week and I'm starting to improve, hence being able to write this. My doctor told me it would lift in a week, I know not all depressions do lift as quickly but they do lift given the right care and treatment.

I think the main thing for me has been to stay calm and do little tasks that I can manage each day as well as resting. Make sure you tell someone how you are truly feeling and there is always the Samaritans who will always be there for you. Try to keep food and fluid intakes up, warm baths can always be soothing, and, if you can manage it, some gentle exercise.

     Again my key word comes up here: don't give up hope. I know how hard it is, but life will and does get better again. It may be a struggle but it becomes more precious, so don't, even at those very low times, give up hope. After all there will always be another sunrise and a new day beginning which brings hope.

CHAPTER TWELVE   A CYCLE OF EPISODES

After finishing the last chapter I've had two more major episodes which I think I need to share with you. I do seem to get a lot but that is because I am a rapid cycler and have more then four episodes a year. The next one started in the Autumn of 2005, I just woke up one day and felt the depression heading my way. I went straight to my GP's who could tell I was suicidal but we couldn't come up with a care package. He then turned up at my house saying the crisis team would be out to see me.

They came that evening, took my tablets away and stated that they would be in to see me everyday. My dad was in hospital for three months during this period for heart surgery, so understandably there was very little family input. Christmas was hell and I just drugged myself up to get through it especially as I wasn't drinking. I slowly got through with the help of the crisis team, until I took a sheer dip down and had to go and see the doctor. She just said I was angry to which I swore back that I was because it was not going away and I stormed out. When I got home I had a phone call from my doctor asking me to go back in and see my previous NHS consultant. During this meeting it was agreed that I needed to go in to hospital for a few days which turned into six weeks.

I ended up in hospital, quite late in the evening, wandering if this was the right thing for me or not. Again I had a clean, albeit sparse, single room and put out the pictures of my two children. That night I awoke to hallucinations of large dogs tearing through my room, and I just ran up the ward in my nightshirt! I got told to put some clothes on and was then talked through what I had seen and given some medication. I had lots of repetitions of this, different hallucinations but all as scary. I met some really lovely girls on this ward and am still in touch with two of them now, and I had visitors from AA but not my family. I fell out with my sister numerous times; mum was very unwell at home whilst trying to take care of the children whilst dad was doing his best.

Each episode I have involves a family upheaval and greatly distresses the children. They get upset whilst it's happening, then angry afterwards. I'm currently getting support and working with family therapy for my son's destructive behaviour: at only eight he is self harming and talks about killing himself. It's also taken a lot of hard work to reassure my daughter and dissipate her anger.

After my first ward round I got told I wasn't under section but if I tried to leave I would be put on one, so what was the difference? It was monotonous in there and I spent most of my time in the smoke room, whilst the staff spent most of their time in the office. You could get one to one time if you asked for it, but it never seemed to be when you needed it due to them being busy. There were never enough beds and a group of patients each night would have to go to another ward to sleep, luckily it wasn't me.

I was put on home leave early though, due to bed shortages, and spent the nights hallucinating and wandering around the empty house which was very scary- when the doctor heard about this I was given my bed back until ward round .From here I was put under the care of the day hospital, but not discharged from the ward so I could still phone the ward if I had any problems. The day hospital was very good and I attended it religiously, it built my confidence back up and lifted my spirits. I had to have community psychiatric assessment before I left, which my sister attended. There was a senior occupational therapist and psychiatric community nurses, one

Lorraine Blackburn

of whom was to be mine, Julie; it all sounded like a good package but we had been let down before and this time they said I had to give up all private care which I reluctantly did.

I have to say though, since then, the care I've had from Julie has been spot on. She's always there if I needed her, understanding and always full of advice. She's a direct link to my doctor, so we can sort out my drugs which we're trying to come down on, even finding the latest research on my sleeping tablet which has been making me have night wanderings and incontinence. This is where is I get baffled and have frustrating days –I know I have an illness and I'm on shed loads of medication but there is no cure, just the illness and the side affects of the drugs. However, I have to remember, in between times, I'm well and lead a reluctantly normal life.

ALIVE WITH BIPOLAR

Over the past year I've been riding an undulating wave, not hitting any where really high or low, but just hovering in those spaces. I did need the home treatment team for a while but I lifted quite quickly out of that low on my own.

My last biggest episode was over this new year just past. I developed diarrhoea and vomiting for about eleven days and either couldn't keep my drugs down or couldn't face taking them, not making any difference having them. So I started to hallucinate. I could hear water splashing nearly all the time in either ear. There were creatures and men in strange suits instead of plant pots and doors; and I kept wandering round not knowing where I was going. I stayed at my mum and dad's during a lot of this and they looked after the children. We then decided to try a night at home; I spent most off it sending odd texts and phone calls to people thinking I was trapped. But finally I was trying to make calls to people and asking them to take my son out of Portsmouth to keep him safe. By this point I had no idea about taking any of my drugs.

My daughter was in floods of tears so she phoned my mum at around ten thirty and my mum came round and got me off to sleep on the futon .Apparently my children where distraught and didn't know what to do; they are only eight and ten years old. The next day I was still completely phased by my drugs and my mum spent ages trying to sort them out with me. I felt confused and was still hallucinating. I tried to phone the out of hour's team for help but I just couldn't find the number, even though I was quite often staring at it. Eventually, after the weekend, Julie got through to me and came and visited me on a regular basis and talked to my mum which helped. So I managed to get through that with mum and Julie and without a hospital admission. I've learnt from my mistakes though; I should have contacted my

ALIVE WITH BIPOLAR

GP, or given someone else the crisis number. I've got a care plan as well which I will now be sticking to the fridge door as I forgot about it last time.

I'm through this episode and so are the children (although I've still got the problems with my son) but I know it really frightened them. It took me a while to get back to driving and on my feet properly. It amazes me though how something physical can have such a major effect on mental aspects. I've got a bout of sinusitis at the moment and I even have to be careful of that. It has made me realise though how much I need to rely on my parents for their support and help and I will be eternally grateful for that. It's my mum's love and care at home, and my dad's, which stopped me from being readmitted

I guess I'm still learning about this illness but the main thing is I'm adapting to it and living with it.

CHAPTER THIRTEEN: ANOTHER ENDING

So here I am, two years on since writing my last book. With regards to my bipolar illness I'm out of the last episode and am coming off some of my drugs. Were also trying to establish a care in the community plan, so the next time I have an episode I can have the Eccuvase injection at my mum's, sleep through it there and have a hand with child care. But we're still waiting for my family to meet with my doctor to discus this; I just desperately want to stay out of St James'. I do have to see the NHS psychiatrist next week which I'm not looking forward to. I feel that too many cooks will spoil my broth.

I remain single and plan to stay that way for a while to come. I've got a lot of growing to do and I need time alone to do it. My ex no longer speaks to me and I have no clear understanding as to why, but it will have to stay that way. I am also starting to lose weight, I'm making the effort but I think the drug changes have helped.

Were in are new home and it is great: this is the first time I have had a solid place to live in my adult life and it feels a relief to be settled. My family have all been supportive but I think I will have problems with the publication of my first book. I think the truth hurts sometimes but I said, at the start of book one, no bullshit and that's how it's got to be.

I haven't worked for a few months but I've just offered to start again, one day a week, as I'm missing it and the money. The divorce is going slowly with a lot of struggling over the financial settlement which is very unpleasant, but I have to keep it in the day and hand my higher power over to my solicitor.

Lorraine Blackburn

So how do I feel? Well I'm now feeling positive again and have hope for a peaceful future. Thus the message for anyone suffering is keep it in the day, and life will improve, you can have a future. We can all survive and this can be seen in my story.

For those of you who have mental health issues in episodes, like me, just try and manage them at the time the best you can. Ask for help, be honest, and remember there is a light at the end of the tunnel, which you will reach. When I reach that end I'm brightened, as if by the northern lights, with such extremes of colours and brightness, whilst the fog lifts and I can see clearly again. It's a change from being possessed, to immense freedom and tranquillity. Most of all never give up, let there always be a firm place in your mind for hope-never let go.

ALIVE WITH BIPOLAR

I've learnt more about my illness and I am the expert to judge it when another episode is happening, and my doctor now trusts in me to do that. I know when I need to cut activities and commitments down. I also know when I need peace and quiet around me, but I do find it hard when there are others around me who don't understand this. I hope so much that these books do become teaching tools as the manageability of my illness would be so much easier if their was a common and fuller understanding. I would walk around with a plaster on my leg saying bipolar episode if I could but I know it wouldn't make any difference. So I'm doing what I can and spreading the word: we are individuals with normal needs and desires, we can give a lot back, and we deserve respect and understanding as much as the next person. I live and I hope. I think my psychiatrist summed it up when he said at my last consultation 'I think your actually going to live

Lorraine Blackburn

Lorraine- it was a close thing!' And I won't just live; I will take on life!

www.ingramcontent.com/pod-product-compliance
Ingram Content Group UK Ltd.
Pitfield, Milton Keynes, MK11 3LW, UK
UKHW041412180426
11947UKWH00007B/89